HOW TO BECOME A GENIUS AND EXPERT IN ANY SUBJECT WITH ACCELERATED LEARNING

HARVEY SEGLER

Want to be productive, healthier and more successful?...

Visit >>> www.ProjectSuperPerformance.com <<< to get free tips about healthy foods, productivity strategies and other nice tricks for a happier, better and more productive life.

At the moment you can get a FREE download of:

"33.5 Power Habits That Will Change Your Life"

But hurry up, the book will not be there forever!

Visit This Website And Download It Now! 100% Free! What Do You Have To Lose?! JustType:

"ProjectSuperPerformance.com"

In Your Search Bar!

If you don't want the book, read the blog which can teach you who wants to be a super performer at work, as a parent, in school or maybe as an athlete how to be just that.

Introduction Chapter

There you are, sitting in front of your laptop again, straining to get through another how to video, or trying to break through a tedious article. All you want to do is learn more about a simple little topic, but it seems that every time you try to learn more about it, or anything else for that matter, nothing will stick.

This is especially annoying when you are trying to learn things that are meant to better your life. Whether it be for your job, for your life skills, or just for general knowledge, it is really hard to keep new knowledge in your head when you are already trying to keep your day in order.

But how do all of those people in the magazines do it? You ask yourself. You talk to the people that you work with, or your friends that you pass in the store. They all seem to be learning and progressing in life, but you, you seem stuck.

That makes it all the more difficult when you are trying to get through you day, and everything seems to be holding you back. You've tried everything. Learning just doesn't seem to come easy to you anymore, and the whole concept of it just seems to be overwhelming.

Don't get discouraged. When you are able to learn effectively, knowledge, facts, and anything else that you need to learn are going to fill your mind. Then you are going to gain and retain knowledge better than ever.

The key here is to learn how to learn. There is an art to it, and when you are able to master that art, you are able to learn in a way that will last a lifetime. Many people don't realize that they have the ability to learn. They think that it is either something that they have or don't.

That couldn't be further from the truth, and you can learn how to learn like a genius. In no time at all, you are going to be able to think like a genius/expert. There won't be anything holding you back, and you are going to be that person that everyone thinks of as the person who knows what to do.

So what are you waiting for? There is a whole world of knowledge out there that is just waiting for you to dive in and absorb. You are never going to view knowledge the same way again.

♥ **Copyright 2015 by Harvey Segler - All rights reserved.**

This document is geared towards providing exact and reliable information in regards to the topic and issue covered. The publication is sold with the idea that the publisher is not required to render accounting, officially permitted, or otherwise, qualified services. If advice is necessary, legal or professional, a practiced individual in the profession should be ordered.

- From a Declaration of Principles which was accepted and approved equally by a Committee of the American Bar Association and a Committee of Publishers and Associations.

In no way is it legal to reproduce, duplicate, or transmit any part of this document in either electronic means or in printed format. Recording of this publication is strictly prohibited and any storage of this document is not allowed unless with written permission from the publisher. All rights reserved.

The information provided herein is stated to be truthful and consistent, in that any liability, in terms of inattention or otherwise, by any usage or abuse of any policies, processes, or directions contained within is the solitary and utter responsibility of the recipient reader. Under no circumstances will any legal responsibility or blame be held against the publisher for any reparation, damages, or monetary loss due to the information herein, either directly or indirectly.

Respective authors own all copyrights not held by the publisher.

The information herein is offered for informational purposes solely, and is universal as so. The presentation of the information is without contract or any type of guarantee assurance.

The trademarks that are used are without any consent, and the publication of the trademark is without permission or backing by the trademark owner. All trademarks and brands within this book are for clarifying purposes only and are the owned by the owners themselves, not affiliated with this document.

Table Of Contents

INTRODUCTION CHAPTER

CHAPTER 1 – THE MINDSET OF A GENIUS

CHAPTER 2 – SPEED READING

CHAPTER 3 – CUTTING THE LEARNING CURVE

CHAPTER 4 – LEARNING FOR THE LONG RUN: THE ART OF RETENTION

CHAPTER 5 – TURNING IT UP AND TUNING IT OUT

CHAPTER 6 – A GENIUS IN THE REAL WORLD

CHAPTER 7 – MAKING TIME TO LEARN

CHAPTER 8 – APPLYING LEARNING TO YOUR OWN LIFE: THE 5 STEPS FOR SUCCESS

CHAPTER 9 – WORKING THE PLAN

CHAPTER 10 – THE LEARNING HOUR: DISSECTED

FREE BONUS

PREVIEW FROM "POSITIVE THINKING"

Chapter 1 – The Mindset of a Genius

I want you to close your eyes for a minute, and picture in your mind a genius. Think of who comes to mind, and think about the extra things that come to your mind when you think of that person.

Odds are, you thought of someone like Albert Einstein or Steven Hawking. Sure, there may have been some other names that flashed through your mind, but if you were to hear the word 'genius' you are likely to think of Albert Einstein as one of the top 3 people.

Let's take a look at this a little further for a second. What is it about him that you are thinking? Are you thinking of him as a teacher? As a scientist? Or perhaps you are thinking of him as that man with the funny hair that we are so used to seeing in our books.

But did you think of him as a learner? Probably not. When we think of the word 'genius' many of us assume that it is a person who is smart and capable, and one that already knows what is going on in the world and how to handle themselves.

Few people think of a person that needs to learn, or a person that is trying to learn new things. Now, I want to clear something up, when you are a genius, or in the genius mindset, you don't need to know everything.

In fact, you don't need to know anything to have the genius mindset. There is a mind that a genius has, and it has nothing to do with knowledge. What a person with the genius mindset has is the ability to learn, and that is what we are going to look at further in the chapters to come.

There are a lot of simple tips that you can utilize that will help you learn how to learn. It does sound funny when you put it like that, but it's true. Everything that you think you know about the concept of learning, you need to forget, and embrace a new way of doing things.

Don't ever assume that there is just one way to learn, and don't hang on to the patterns of learning that you have used in the past. Clearly, those methods aren't working for you right now. They may have worked for you in the past, and they may work for you now, but unless you know for sure that they are going to work tomorrow, don't assume.

You need to know for sure what does work, and that in itself is a genius mindset. You need to know that there is a method to learning, and you need to learn what that method is for you. There is no right and wrong way to learn, it is all personal to you.

But I try to learn, but I don't think that anything will stick.

This is a common problem that a lot of people face. They want to learn, but they find that they aren't able to hang on to anything that they learn. No matter how hard they try, it seems as though everything goes in one ear and back out the other.

They try to learn how they did when they were in school, but that doesn't seem to make a difference to you now. Not to mention the fact when you do need something explained, it is really hard to ask for help, because you don't want anyone to think that you aren't smart or that you are silly.

I am telling you right now you need to get over that feeling. There isn't anything at all wrong with asking for help, and it doesn't make you dumb or foolish if you need to have something explained differently or in a better way.

When you are learning to view life as a genius does, you need to get over the fear of other people, and have the confidence to learn... and ask for things to be taught to you.

The mark of a true genius is to know when to ask for help.

Don't ever be ashamed about asking for help, or asking that someone explains something to you. There are all kinds of people on this planet, and there are people that know some things that other people don't know.

When you are in the process of learning like a genius, you need to realize that there isn't anyone on this planet that is smarter than you, they just know different things than you do.

The whole point of society and growing as a group, is to learn together, then pass on knowledge to each other. It doesn't do much good for anyone to make fun of each other if you don't know how to do something, or to put up with people that make fun of you if you don't know something.

Another thing you need to keep in mind is "like attracts like".

There is a point where this does go beyond the concept of learning and merges into the concept of coexisting. We can't all know everything, and if we live in a way that allows us to grow and help each other, then we will all make it.

What this all really comes down to is confidence. Be ok with being yourself, and be ok with your own learning style. You aren't foolish, and you aren't dumb for learning things in a certain way. What is important is that you find out what your own learning style is, and you pursue your knowledge acquisition in that light.

When you are able to embrace your own personal learning style, you are able to learn things in a way that is entirely suited to you, and you will find that your learning is going to grow by leaps and bounds.

What you learn you will be able to retain, and you are going to learn things that will stick with you.

Chapter 2 – Speed Reading

For some, the concept of learning fills them with a lot of excitement. People want to jump in and learn right off, and they want to be able to absorb and retain and expand.

For others, they want to learn, but it doesn't come easy to them. This shouldn't be too surprising of a concept… we all know that there are kids who struggle in school, and there are those that we work with that seem to have a really difficult time learning the company policies and how to do their jobs.

Maybe you are one of those people that has a hard time learning how to do things, and you don't even know what to do when it comes to learning. You know that you want to learn how to do things, but it seems to take so long.

Whether that be taking out an instruction manual, downloading a new book on how to do something, or finding articles about it online, reading seems to be something that we have to do if we want to learn something new.

Sure, there are those videos that we can watch to learn, but in all honesty, it is a fact that people learn better as a whole if they are able to read something for themselves rather than watching a video.

We all want that quick fix way of learning, but did you know one of the fastest ways to learn is to read? It may be surprising, but it's true. Reading is an amazing way to learn.

Now, I'm not saying that films, YouTube clips, or podcasts are bad ways of learning... but I do think reading is a lot better.

Why, you ask?

The answer is simple, and it lies in the matter of focus. When you are reading something, you are reading it in the silence of your brain, and you are able to quiet your mind from other distractions and focus on what you are reading.

So if learning is so much better of a way to learn, is there a way to be more effective at reading? As a matter of fact, there is. The answer comes in speed... that is, how fast you are able to read something.

Think about it: what if you learned a way to read a book 300% faster than you would under normal circumstances. Imagine how much more information you could absorb in a shorter amount of time, and imagine how you can cut your learning curve.

I know it sounds intimidating, but it is entirely possible. The learning curve is something that holds a lot of people back when it comes to how they pick up on new things, and it largely discourages people from trying to learn new things.

If you are able to master the art of speed reading, you are able to learn things a lot faster than you ever thought possible, and you will be able to achieve success even sooner.

Ok, so I want to learn how to speed read, but how do I learn how to do something that I have always done even faster?

There are simple tips and tricks that you can follow that will help you learn how to pick up on this trait, and once you learn, you won't have an issue with it at all.

The first thing you want to keep an eye on is efficiency. You want to make sure that you don't read any unnecessary text. Once you learn how to do that, you will save a lot of time.

It does take practice to learn what text is necessary and what is irrelevant, but with time, you are going to master this concept. Some irrelevant things are easy to identify, such as the reviews written in the book to give the book and the author a higher authority, and a few other things.

However, do not make the mistake of skipping the introduction.

Why?

The answer is simple. The author needs to catch your interest in the introduction, and will often place a lot of helpful information there.

Now, in the next chapter, let's take a look at the steps you can take that will help you become a faster reader. These are things that you can start doing today, and things that you need to work on over time to master.

Don't be discouraged if you can't do it at first, some things take time.

Chapter 3 – Cutting the Learning Curve

There is this thing that everyone has... what it technically is... is the time it takes to learn something. This is called the learning curve, and it is a major point of stress or achievement for people, depending on who you are and what your own particular style is.

As we saw in the last chapter, reading has a major effect on your learning curve, and it is important to learn how to speed read in order to cut down on that curve.

Step 1

The first thing that you need to do when you are learning how to speed read, is to figure out what your current pace is, so you know where you need to improve. It is impossible to know where you need to be if you don't know where you are right now, so for the first step, we need to look at what your current pace is.

You want to read for a bit longer time. Maybe 10-15 pages is enough. But it could be a bit frustrating (and slow) counting 3000+ words... So this is what you want to do:

1. Grab a book, fiction preferable.

2. Count the amount of words on 10 lines

3. Divide all those words with 10 and you will have the average number of words per line

4. Now, count the amount of lines on about three pages and divide it with three, that is the average number of lines per page.

5. Multiply the numbers (words per line x lines per page) and you will have the average amount of words per page.

6. Take the time while reading 10-15 pages. Multiply the amount of pages with the average number of words per page.

7. Divide that last number with the number of minutes it took for you reading those pages

8. DONE! That is the number of words you read per minute. Do not forget to wright it down

Pro tip: You can also take a text from the internet and copy it into microsoft word so you don't need to count the words (it should show the amount of words at the bottom), but be sure to print it out so you can also use it for step 3

Now! The fun part, learning.

Step 2

So when we read, our eyes are not moving with consistent pace. They are actually jumping and taking snapshots. They are jumping from word to word, and sometimes they are actually jumping backwards. So if we could cancel that out we have already made a huge advancement. How do you do it? Do you need some fancy $35.000 laser surgery? NO! The only thing you need is your finger or a pen. Put the pen or your finger right under the text line and then, you just want to follow the text while reading. This step is so easy but will make a real difference on your reading pace. This will teach your eyes to follow a straight line and not jumping, especially not backwards. You will have to practice this for some minutes before continuing.

Firstly, read in the same pace as usually but while underlining. Do this for about 5 min. Then try to speed up a bit, and do that for 5 more minutes. Lastly, read some minutes as fast as you could, of course still underlining.

Step 3

When you are looking at something, lets say this line:

_____

When you are looking at it you are still seeing things around it, like these words. This is your peripheral vision and it allows you seeing things without focusing at them. Most of us do not take advantage of this when we read, but you could and should. If you do not take in this forthcoming tip you will lose about 50% of your vision... Too much of a loss, don't you think? The solution is just as easy as the one in "Step 2". Instead of putting your pen under the first word of each line you want to start 2 or 3 words in. And also you want to stop that pen 2-3 words from the end of each line. This is a skill and you will have to practice. Start with one word from the start and the end and try to read like this for a couple of minutes. Then move on to 2 words and if you master that, 3 words will be the last and final step.

The 3 words step is a bit harder and you may have to practice for some extra minutes.

At the beginning of these steps, you may have a hard time putting the pen on the right place. So you could draw a line to help yourself. Obviously you should not do this in a book you want to look like new, but maybe on some papers or an old letter.

Step 4

It is time for measurement, again. Do exactly as we did in step one, but this time you read in the new, faster and more time efficient way. Write down that new number. Did you already achieve 300%? if you did, fantastic! If not, you will just have to practice more. Even if you did or did not, move on to step 5.

Step 5

Now. Do what you have learned in step 2 and 3 over and over again. More practice = faster reading. And take the time while reading. You want to have a time goal, lets say 900 words in a minute. That is 15 words/second. Pretty hard? Yes. But setting that goal will help you achieve higher speed. Don't just set a goal in your mind, write it down!! This will help you really se your goal and achieve it.

But what does all of this have to do with learning?

The biggest lesson you are trying to learn with your speed reading is to focus. There is a lot of benefits to the art of focus, and you are going see that you can retain a lot better when you are focused.

That is one of the biggest issues a lot of people have with learning today. They are not focused on what they are doing, and they don't actually read. It is as though they are staring at the words on the screen, but they aren't actually getting any of them.

This is what you need to break out of, and what you need to be aware of when you are speed reading. Read quickly, sharpen your skills so you are reading through your words faster, but also make sure you are retaining them.

How do I know if I am retaining them if I don't have to use the information right away?

A good way to ensure that you are retaining what you are reading is to have little mini quizzes that you look over when you are finished with your reading. Perhaps you want to make a list of questions that you need to know the answer to by the time you reach the end of the section.

Of course, this is going to take time to perfect, but you need to sharpen your skill in this area if you want to make sure that you are effectively learning. If you don't, then you are going to fall victim to the trap of reading but not retaining, and that is nothing more than a waste of your time.

An effective learner knows the value of time.

If you want to master the art of learning, you need to learn the value of time. A person that knows the value of time is a person that knows how to use it effectively, and will make the most out of what they have.

If you don't know the value of the time that you have, then you won't be using it properly, and you will find that you waste a lot of time. There is nothing worse in this day than wasting time.

You know that you only have so much of it, and while you want to enjoy the process of learning, you also want to be able to keep what you learn. There is little point to taking the time and making the effort of learning how to do something, then forgetting it as soon as you close the book.

I want you to be able to read something, and keep it. Don't worry about how many fine details you are able to remember at first, what is important is the main points. You will find in your speed reading that you are really just learning to pick out the main point of what the author is saying.

When you realize that is what you are trying to do, it becomes that much easier to speed read, as you are able to see what you need to learn, and you are able to retain it better.

Chapter 4 – Learning for the Long Run: The Art of Retention

As we saw in the last chapter, it doesn't do you a lot of good if you are reading and forgetting. No, you are learning to think like a genius. Now, many people assume that a genius is able to immediately know what is going on, or that they are able to understand whatever it is that they are reading.

Let me assure you, this isn't the case. Many people, genius or not, don't understand what they read the first time around. Sure, they are able to piece some things together, or they are able to reread it and find out what they are supposed to learn, but you need to realize that just because you don't understand something the first time, that doesn't mean that you won't understand it in the long run.

Sometimes you need to take a step back and read the same passage again. There isn't anything wrong with reading something two or three times in order to grasp a full understanding of it. What is important is that you do have that understanding before you move on with your learning.

Use what learning style works for you.

There are thousands of people on this planet, and there are just as many ways to learn things. Don't assume that there is just one way to learn something, and that you are learning it wrong if you learn in a way that is different from other people that you know.

Some people learn by doing, and some people learn by reading. Then there are those that learn by taking notes. For still others, they find that they are able to learn best when they read something out loud.

When you are learning, you need to find what works for you, and go with that method. Even if it means that you need to learn in a different way for different topics. What I mean by that is that you may learn to cook by doing, and you may learn to draw by reading.

My point is that there isn't a wrong way to learn, and what works for you is what you need to do, or you aren't going to learn effectively, and that means you are likely to forget what you have learned.

Another thing that you need to keep in mind is that no one can tell you what your learning style is. You need to find that out for yourself, and not worry about if that is what other people are doing or not.

When you know what works for you, you can build your confidence on that. Don't worry about what other people think of your learning style, and don't worry about whether or not it is how other people are learning.

Find that stand out point that makes a point 'click'.

We all have our own unique learning styles, we have learned that much, but we also need to learn that point in which things just seem to stick with us. Some of us need to make a point of doing something one way, others need to find something about it to help them remember how to do it.

This can go hand in hand with the thought process that you need to find your own learning style, but it does go a bit beyond that with the idea that you need to make a point to find something unique about the topic to make it stick with you.

To better clarify what I am talking about, think about it this way: when you meet someone new, if you aren't good with names, it is likely that you try to find something about them that will help you remember their name.

It is a common trick that a lot of experts recommend you try to help you remember a new face. And what is remarkable about this is that it works, really well for a lot of people, too.

You want to make a point of implementing this learning style into whatever it is you are trying to learn. It works for all kinds of things, whether it be a lesson of some kind, or if it is a new skill you are trying to learn.

No matter what the case may be, you need to learn how to keep things in your mind. Our minds are constantly changing and growing, and it isn't at all uncommon for them to discard information that we no longer find necessary.

It is almost a self-cleaning mechanism that makes it easier to function in life, but at the same time it can also make it difficult to keep new things in your mind. This is why our minds tend to make a note of things that are a bigger deal to us than things that aren't.

It is for this reason that you often more likely to remember things that are embarrassing than things that are just mundane and ordinary. When you are learning like a genius, you learn to view the world through eyes that are watching for opportunity, and you are able to keep a hold of your information a lot better.

Chapter 5 – Turning it Up and Tuning it Out

Let's be realistic here. No matter how much you would like to, it just isn't realistic for you to be in a quiet classroom to learn everything. There are so many things that need to be learned on the run, and it is hard to find the peace and quiet to learn them.

This is the hardest part of learning for most people. They are able to pick a topic to learn about, but when it comes down to the nitty gritty of sitting still and learning, it just doesn't happen.

Now, this could be for a number of reasons. You might try to sit down and learn, but there is noise and other distractions that manage to creep in that make it difficult to learn.

Or, you may have every intention to sit down and learn about a certain topic, but you find as soon as you get something like the internet involved, there is way too many other things that pop up that make it nearly impossible for you to stay on topic and learn about what you intended to learn.

But I don't have a problem with that, I have a problem with absorbing what I am reading.

This is yet another common problem that many people run into. Sure, they are able to get to where they need to be. They are able to get the peace and quiet while they are reading about it, but they have a really hard time grasping what they are reading.

You may be dealing with this yourself. You sit in front of a page or a screen and you read and reread, but it just doesn't seem to stick. In the past chapters, we have looked at great ways to find your learning style, but that may not cure this problem.

In order to solve this sort of issue, you need to clear your mind and pay attention. This isn't so much an issue of external distractions as it is one of internal distractions.

Your thoughts play a major role in this sort of thing. You need to control them, and make them focus on what you are learning. Don't worry, the good news is that this is a common problem with a common solution.

At first, it is nothing more than a conscious effort to pay attention and learn. If you really have a difficult time with even that, then go for the method of keeping notes. That is the most surefire way of ensuring that you are paying attention.

When you know that you need to write down the main points, then you are sure to pay attention to what you are reading. You may need to do this all the while, whenever you learn, but there are those that are able to break out of it and focus.

We have a lot more power over our own thoughts than most people like to admit. It is a lot easier to push it off on our brains or as an issue that we can't get around, but we actually can control our thoughts in a number of ways.

Next time you sit down to read something, close your eyes, take a few deep breaths, and clear your mind. It doesn't matter if you need to do this in public or not, if you need to do it, then you should.

You are going to find that you keep your knowledge a lot easier when you do this, so don't skip this step, and keep your confidence up so you actually do it. It is important that put these things into practice, even if you don't feel confident doing them at first.

We are also very trainable as people, and if we do things that we aren't comfortable with at first, it isn't long before we do become comfortable with them, and they are just second nature to us.

Gaining control of your thoughts is no exception, and you are going to find that you are able to focus a lot better, and retain a lot better than you ever thought possible.

Chapter 6 – A Genius in the Real World

You will find that becoming a genius in the real world is going to have its challenges. There are things that are easy to accomplish, which, ironically, are the things that we listed in this book.

Then, there are the things that are harder to accomplish, and those two things in particular are: (1) people... the world as a whole, and (2) you... working against yourself. You will find that on the outset of this endeavor, you are going to be your own worst enemy.

You are going to be the one standing in your own way as you try to work around your bad habits, and as you try to develop new ones. Then, there are your own doubts, these will plague you for a long time.

Now, don't get discouraged, they will go away, especially if you work at keeping them down and developing confidence. What you do need to do is stay consistent. Don't ever let yourself put yourself down, and don't think things about yourself that will slow you down.

There isn't any reason to be arrogant, but at the same time, you can't ever put yourself down. You aren't going to get anywhere if you live a life that holds yourself back.

But then there is the second on the list, and that is other people. Yes, it is true that you are the first and hardest being to get around when you are working on your learning curve and becoming a better learner, but after you break out of that, you are going to find that other people come in to play, and they are not so nice.

These people are the ones that can't stand to see someone else be successful, and they will do what they can to hold you back. It is a cruel fact of nature, and you are going to have to deal with it. There isn't anything that you can do about it, but you can work around it.

Don't let other people get you down, and don't put yourself down, either. When you break out of that kind of thinking, and when you refuse to let others bring you down, then you are going to be a real genius.

You are more capable than you think, and you are more than able to be that genius that you want to be. Don't let anyone bring you down and make the most of every opportunity you have to learn.

Once you are able to view this life as a gift, and every learning experience as an opportunity to further yourself in this life, and to make the most out of what you have, you will be an even bigger genius than anyone that came to mind when you thought of the person in chapter 1.

So what are going waiting for? You can do whatever you set your mind to, so don't ever let anyone hold you back, you got this

Chapter 7 – Making Time to Learn

It is no secret that we all live very busy lives. Many people who want to learn new things or better themselves often stay stuck in the same rut in their life because they just feel like they don't have the time to learn something new.

It can be really intimidating to take on a new challenge. Whether that be losing weight, changing jobs or where you live, learning a new skill, or even just taking on a hobby... it can feel crushing if you are already stretched thin in your schedule.

So what can you do to get around this? The answer to that question is easier than you might think.

Use the time that you have.

It doesn't matter how much time you have in your day to dedicate to learning this new skill... it might be ten minutes for some, it might be an hour for other people, but if you really want to learn something new, and you are willing to set aside the time in your day to learn it, work with what you have.

You will be surprised at how much you can learn in a short amount of time when you are willing to focus your mind on that.

Debunking the 10,000 hour rule.

There are people in this world who are superstars. We all know this. They are great at what they do, in fact, they are the champions of the world.

A study was done of these athletes and superstars trying to determine how long it takes to get to that level of achievement. Through tests and other studying of these people, it has been determined that it takes thousands of hours to get to that level of performance. Of course that is not a surprise, and it is rather discouraging to those that just want to learn how to do something.

That is where we come in. Sure, it does take thousands of hours if you want to be the best in the world at something, but the truth of the matter is that not many of us want to be champions at a given activity.

You might want to learn how to cook fine culinary creations, or perhaps you want to learn Chinese. These are wonderful goals to have, but the odds that you want to be the best chef in the whole world or teach Chinese to children in China are pretty slim. For those of us that are just trying to learn a new skill, the 10,000 hour 'rule' isn't a rule at all.

It is a myth that the shorter amount of time you spend on something in a day, then longer it will take you to learn it.

If you focus on what you want to learn, you can learn it in a short amount of time, even if you only have a few minutes a day to spend on that subject.

Chapter 8 – Applying Learning to Your Own Life: The 5 Steps for Success

While we have already looked at a lot of different tips and tricks that you can use that will help you in your learning process, let's take it a step further and look at something a little more solid.

You get the concept, you know what you want to learn, but now you sit there, spinning your wheels so to speak.

"How can I apply this to my own life, and learn the things that I want to learn on my limited schedule?" You ask yourself. Don't worry, that is a very common question, and it is one that can be worked around. Yes, it does take time and effort for you to learn what you want to learn, but with these steps you are going to get there in no time at all.

Step 1 – Decide what your goal actually is.

This is a universal step, and it applies to anything that you could ever want to learn. You need to know what it is you want to get out of an activity, and what your end goal is with this activity.

That goes for all activities, whether it is a mental thing that you want to learn, or some sort of motor skill such as riding a bike or skydiving. Remember, once you have your eyes set on something, you have a target to shoot for.

Once you have what you want in mind, you are able to look for ways to reach that goal, no matter what it is. This is why it is important to pick a specific goal. If you are just looking at a generalized topic you are going to get bogged down with all kinds of information that you don't necessarily need.

Now, if you pick something that is specific, for example, if you decide you want to be a pastry chef versus someone who cooks, then you are naturally going to look for ways to make your skill better. You will be drawn to sections in bookstores that are on the topic of your choice, and you will want to watch programs that are about what you want.

If you want to be a pastry chef you aren't going to care how to marinate a steak, so pick your practice early on, and gravitate towards the things that are going to get you there.

Remember, when you are learning anything new, that you don't want to be too specific in your target goal. There is a fine line between knowing what you want and going for it, and having just one circumstance in mind that you hope pans out.

For example, instead of thinking "I want to have a conversation with a particular person in their native language", it is better to think, "I want to be able to easily converse with a foreign person in their own language".

And another thing to keep in mind is that the first few hours of learning anything is frustrating, but you can't give up. These hours may feel like an eternity now, but the more time you spend doing something, the easier it is going to be to do it.

Step 2 – Picking apart a skill.

When we think of a goal that we want to achieve, we tend to categorize it in ways that we shouldn't. For example, we tend to think of things such as playing a sport, or writing a book, or cooking to be skills, but they aren't really skills at all.

Playing a sport is a worthy goal to have, but in and of itself, it is not a skill. Running, catching, aiming, an understanding of physics, etc... these are all skills that add up to playing a sport. So, if you are trying to learn a sport, you are going to need to practice these skills in order to achieve your goal.

This is why it is important to hone in on a particular goal. If you know what you want, then you will be able to better analyze how you want to reach that goal. You may be surprised to learn that most of the major things we as people want to learn in life, are really composed of three or four smaller skills that need to be practiced.

But how do you know what these skills are? Well, that is something that is going to take a bit of time and research. You may have to sit down and analyze what you want to be or learn to figure out how to actually achieve it. That is where step three comes in.

Step 3 – Research the skills that you will need for your goal.

You may cringe at the sound of the word 'research'. Who has time for that, after all? We have already mentioned that you don't have all this spare time in a day, so how are you supposed to sit down and read about what you need to learn?

Thankfully, step three is a step that really shouldn't take very long. We are taught that research is supposed to be a lengthy process that takes up all kinds of time and energy, but that doesn't need to be the case at all.

When you are researching what you should learn in order to acquire a new skill, try doing this simple method that will cut down your research time drastically:

Go to the library, and check out five or six books on the topic that you want to learn. Be specific. Again, if you are wanting to be a pastry chef, then check out books on that specific genre, don't check out books that are about cooking in general. Youtube videos, blogs, movies, online courses - all sorts of information resources is great as well.

Next, take your books home, sit down, and skim them. Don't waste time reading them cover to cover, but rather, flip through them and see what the three or four major things are that they have in common.

These are going to be the skills that you need to practice in order to learn what you are trying to learn.

It really is as simple as that. Then, once you have determined what skills you need to learn, you are going to be a lot better able to get out there and pick up on those skills than you would be wasting time reading about what you want to learn.

There is a bit of a problem in the world today, and with the society that we are a part of. We are a very academic society, and many people hold learning in high regard, but then learning tends to take a turn for the worst, and we make a mistake.

We waste way too much time when we are researching. Yes, when authors put together books on topics they want to make sure they give their readers everything that they want, but if we really come down to it, we spend a lot of time reading things that aren't necessary to the skill that we are trying to learn.

If you want to make the most of the time that you spend learning something, you need to make sure you aren't wasting even a minute of that time. The more time spent messing around, the less time you have to spend on the actual practice.

We have said time and time again, practice makes perfect, and when you are learning anything, the more hands on time you have, the sooner you are going to learn the skill that you want to learn. Anyone can read about a skill, hobby, or topic, but if you want to make it your own, you need to get your nose out of the book, and start doing it.

Step 4 – Prepare your work environment.

Whenever you are learning a new skill, it is important that you have an environment that makes it easy to learn. Find an area that you can practice your skill and not be distracted. The more distractions you have, the harder it is going to be to learn a new skill. This is crucial.

Many people try to multi-task. They feel that they don't have the time to learn a new skill as is, so they try to get other things done while they are learning. This <u>may</u> be ok when you are past the initial phases of learning a skill, but in the early stages, it is important that you are focused on the still at hand, and free your mind of other distractions.

You may need to shut off the computer and the television, you might need to turn off your phone. You might need to be alone. There are all kinds of different things that you might need to do in order to learn what you are trying to learn, but you have got to do it.

Another thing to keep in mind is that you should make it easy to learn your new skill. What we mean by that is… keep it out in the open. If you want to learn how to draw, don't bury your book and pencils in the bottom of your drawer.

Set them out on your desk so you see them and you make an effort to get to them in your day. The first few hours of learning anything new are going to be plenty frustrating enough as it is, so do what you can on the outset to make it as smooth and pain free as possible.

Don't make learning a chore, and don't ever force yourself into what you want to do. Do what you need to do to make it easy for yourself. We learn the best when we are at ease and enjoying what we are doing. Pressure might help you get something done fast, but relaxation is what is going to help you get it done well.

You are trying to learn a new skill that you will carry with you for the rest of your life. You don't want that to be a bad memory of something that you hated, you want it to be fun and enjoyable. It has been said that no one has the most fun when they completed a project, they have fun when they are working on it.

Yes, you want to be there today, you want to be what you want to be right now, but you should take the time to enjoy the work, and keep track of how far you are coming. There is nothing wrong with the process of something, so make the most of it.

Step 5 – Commit to spending 20 hours on learning something.

Many people shrink back when they hear the word 'commit', but don't worry, this is going to be painless, and it is for your own good. There are few things worse in life than wasting your time, so that is something you ought to avoid at all cost, and that is the point of this time line commitment.

Before you set out to learn anything, commit to twenty hours of practice for this skill. This is really a commitment that is meant to test yourself on how serious you are on learning the skill.

Many people shy away at the thought of spending 20 hours doing something, but in truth, you can become really good at something in that amount of time. Sure, everyone learns at their own pace, and everyone learns differently, but if you are dedicated to learning something, and you set aside that amount of time out of your life to do it, you will be amazed at how far you come in less than a day's time.

"But when I used to learn things as a kid, it took me days to practice it," you tell yourself. This may be true, but if you really think about it, there were a lot of outside influences that went into those twenty hours that made it seem like it took a lot longer than it really did. Perhaps you didn't even really want to learn what you were learning, or maybe you would have rather been doing other things the entire time.

You have to ask yourself: How many days did you skip practice? How many times did you say you working on it for a full hour, when you really only worked on it for a few minutes?

There are a number of other variables that come into play here, but the truth of the matter is that there are a lot of studies to back up the twenty hour practice. Not only that, if you really think about it, there are a lot of benefits that also come into play when you give yourself a time limit… you can also see how much time you have left before you get to your goal.

No matter how long you are actually working on something, it is going to feel like it is taking you a lot longer to do it than it really is. This idea is that you are going to commit to a timed period so you know for sure the amount of time you are dedicating to a new practice.

Chapter 9 – Working the Plan

As we have mentioned before, there are two different kinds of skills, and these are motor skills and mental skills. The name really says it all when it comes to the difference between the two.

A motor skill is a skill that is physical. It pertains to such things as balance, endurance, and other activities that you do with your body. Mental skills are things such as learning a new language, learning how to do something new, and other activities that have to do with the mind.

It may come as a surprise to you, but we learn mental skills and motor skills differently, and there are things that we can do that will making learning these things easier.

Motor skills.

There are actual studies that show it is <u>easier to learn a motor skill and retain how to do that skill if you practice doing it within 2 hours of going to sleep.</u>

Whether you are taking a nap or going to bed for the day, it doesn't really matter, but if you are trying to pick up on a new motor skill, you should make an effort to practice it close to when you are going to be sleeping.

You can even make an effort to fall asleep shortly after doing it, for example, intentionally take a nap a couple hours after doing a skill, just to help it stay in your mind better.

Put it into practice: tonight, close to when you are going to go to bed, make a deliberate effort to try something that you haven't done before. It doesn't have to be anything major... you can try typing very fast, or drawing a specific figure, or anything like that, then go to bed.

Then, when you get up in the morning, again try to do what you did the night before. You will see a noticeable difference in how well you can do it in the morning than when you went to bed, guaranteed.

Mental learning methods.

There is more flexibility when it comes to mental practice. Different people learn differently, and how you are going to learn depends on your own particular style.

What you need to do to put this kind of learning into practice is find what your best method of learning is, then practice as much as you can using that method. If you are a person that learns better with flash cards, invest in some.

Perhaps you are a person that learns better with taking notes. Find lectures online and take notes as the speaker is talking. Whatever your method is, no matter what it is, do it frequently, and you are going to see how much better you retain the knowledge.

Another thing to keep in mind is that while mental skills are learned differently than motor skills, you are going to get better benefit learning it close to going to sleep.

The 10,000 hour rule and the 20 hour commitment.

The truth of the matter is that you have to take the time to actually learn what you want to learn. There is speed reading, there is accelerated learning, but there is no way around the fact that you have to actually put in the time and effort to do it.

Like we already looked at, it has been said that it takes ten thousand hours to become a professional at something. This is more time than many of us can ever dream of having, so that turns into a real discouragement when you think that you have to spend that much time learning something new.

There is good news, however, in that you don't actually have to spend that amount of time learning anything. As we saw in the five steps to learning, you only have to dedicate twenty hours to learning something if you want to get really good at it.

Now, for many others, this also feels like a lot of time, but you have to remember that you need to be patient. When we think we want to learn something new, we always think of how it will be when we are already good at it. How good we will feel, how awesome everyone around us will think we are, and how complete our lives will then be.

We know what we want, and we want it right now. Who wants to wait to get that good at something? Who wants to have to suffer through all of the frustration and the failures that come with learning anything? Nobody, that's for sure, but then you have to remember that nobody is great at something the first time they start.

That is where the twenty hour rule comes in. There are plenty of studies that show that anyone is a lot better at a skill after they have worked at it for twenty hours. Sure, they may not be an super expert, but they are certainly a lot better at it than when they started.

For many people, getting good enough at something to enjoy it when they do it is all they really want. There aren't many people out there who set out to be the best in the world at a given topic, so why not dedicate the time and effort you need to get good at something?

Remember, if you don't have twenty hours to dedicate to something… or if you don't think that twenty hours is worth dedicating to learning something new, then you should move along with your day and forget about it.

In the grand scheme of things, twenty hours isn't very long when it is compared to having a skill that you can use for the rest of your life, so why not put that amount of time aside?

You need to ask yourself how serious you are about learning, and you if you are really dedicated to picking up on the new skill, you are going to be thrilled with the results.

Chapter 10 – The Learning Hour: Dissected

Let's take a minute now to break down what a learning session actually looks like. You learned the 5 steps that it takes to pick up a new skill, but what do those steps look like all played out?

It is one thing to study something in theory, it is quite another to put that theory into action. If you are serious about learning anything, and it doesn't matter what that is... if you want to learn it in a way that you will actually progress in the skill, then do this, and you will.

Clear out a section of your room and dedicate it to the activity.

That is action step one, and you need to go do it, right now. At this point, we know that you have your skill in mind, and you know for sure what you want to do. You have also committed to spending twenty hours practicing this skill, so get your area ready.

You want your area to be free of distraction. Don't be in earshot of the television, or the computer. Make sure you aren't looking out a window, either. There are all kinds of distractions that manage to creep in through there.

Put away anything visual that will take your mind away from the new skill, and put it all away. If you want to add in anything to this area, add in what will make you focus and press you to practice your skill. These things can be anything:

- Posters of people good at the skill that inspire you
- Inspirational quotes
- Tools you will need for the skill
- Reminders of what you need to focus on learning
- Anything else that will keep you focused and on the task at hand

In addition to these things, keep a timer and a notebook in your area. These are going to be used to help you keep track of the time you are spending on the practice.

Clear your mind.

There is no way you can focus on what you are practicing if you are worried about something. You need to make sure you have everything done and out of your mind before you sit down to practice.

This goes along with getting rid of all distractions. You need to make sure your mind is as clear and focused as the area you set up, or you are going to be wasting your time with trying to learn something that will seem impossible.

Sure, you might have other things that you need to do in a day, but make sure you have a set amount of time that you can dedicate to learning this new skill, worry free. If you need to do it last thing before bed, that's fine, if you need to do it before dinner, that's fine, too.

Whatever it takes for you to clear your mind and focus on what you are trying to learn, do that.

Meditation could be a great way doing this. Maybe that should be the first thing you should learn.

Set your timer for the amount of time you have.

There are two benefits to this. For starters, you can keep track of how long you spend doing the activity. This is going to help you when you feel frustrated or like you aren't getting anywhere on it even though you have been working for 'days'.

Another benefit is that you can work on your project, worry free. You know that you have other things that you need to do, but you also know that you have this amount of time set aside for practice. That can be any amount of time that you need, whatever works for you.

If you want to have a time frame charted out for you, think of it this way: twenty hours is broken up to about 40 minutes per day, every day for a month.

So if you are willing or able to set aside forty minutes a day, you will be at your twenty hours in a single mont. that seems to be pretty fast considering how long you may have thought it was going to take.

Don't have forty minutes all at once? That's fine, too. You are going to spend a certain amount of time *per day*. This can be broken into four, ten minute sessions or two, twenty minute sessions.

The key here is to draw up a formula that works for you, and stick with that formula once you have it drawn.

Use a pen and keep track of your time… and progress.

When you dedicate twenty hours to learning something new, you want to know where you are in your time, so keep your notebook up to date with your time sheet.

When you start working on your practice, set the timer, and write down how long you spend on it each day. It is as simple as that. You will be surprised at how fast the time really does go, especially when you are a few days into it.

Another thing that you are going to want to keep track of is your progress. You will, of course, see this naturally when you are practicing your new skill, but if you jot down your achievements in the notebook, you are going to be able to see even better how far you have come.

Look back at day 1 when your month is up.

Once you have completed the month, take a few minutes and flip back to day one, and see how far you have come. Of course you are going to have your newly acquired skill to show you how far you have come, but there are few things so powerful as being able to look back at day one and see where you were, then look at where you are now.

It really doesn't take too much time to pick up on a new skill, and when you are dedicated to learning and making that skill your own, it becomes even more surprising how fast it goes.

Turn off those lights.

Above all, in your learning, you have to keep in mind that you will learn things better and faster when you practice right before you sleep. This isn't a luxury that everyone can have, and we understand that, but you need to make an effort to do it as much as you can.

Two hours is the most ideal time frame that we recommend you use, but if that is just not possible, then you should aim for four hours at the most. This is a lot more doable for a lot of people that aren't able to make the two hour mark, and there are still incredible results when you are practicing.

The best way to do it is to nap in between sessions, but some people aren't able to fall asleep during the day. This is, of course, remedied by practicing at night, as everyone is able to sleep for the night when they finally go to bed. What you need to do is find what works for you, but is as close to these steps as possible.

There are always going to be exceptions and variations in everything that you do, so all you can do is your best. Everyone has a busy life, and everyone is wanting to learn and become better than they are. What we are promising is that you can do that if you are willing to put in the time to do it.

Don't sweat the small things, skim books for the big things, and set aside a special place for you to be able to focus. If you do these things, you are going to pick up on any skill that you set your mind to, and you are going to see the results that you want to see.

So what are you waiting for? Get ready to learn... and think... like a real expert and genius.

Conclusion

Thank you for downloading this book!

I would call this the key to knowledge and learning, but really, you didn't need me to have that, as that is what our own brains are. When you are able to unleash your shyness, and rein in your thoughts, great things not only can happen, they will.

You need to have the confidence that you can learn, and you need to have the attitude of a genius and an expert. Yes, it is really easy to assume that you can't do it, or that it won't work out for you, but that isn't what being a genius is about, and that is no attitude to have if you are going to break out of this thought process and grow in your own life.

I am not saying that it isn't going to be hard, any new habit is hard when we are first learning how to do it, but what I am saying is that it is going to be worth your time and efforts, and that you will be glad that you took the time to follow through on this.

Remember that in this world we live in, there are going to be people that are for us, and there are always going to be those people that are jealous and who try to put us down. Be confident in your knowledge, and be confident in your abilities.

Don't let anyone put you down, and don't get into petty arguments, you are capable, and you are able to be confident in your own quiet genius.

Don't ever assume that you are too much of anything to be unable to learn, and there is a genius inside of all of us, so don't be afraid to let your knowledge and capabilities shine!

<u>Finally</u>, if you enjoyed this book, then I'd like to ask you for a favor, would you be kind enough to leave a review for this book on Amazon? It'd be greatly appreciated! I am a self published author and I would love to hear you thoughts! If the review is critical, please provide me with things you think I should change. This way I can import the book. Thanks.

Visit: www.amazon.com//dp/B0161L2WES

to leave a review for this book on Amazon!

And do not forget to visit the website ProjectSuperPerformance.com! Free and fantastic content about a lot of different things! How to lose weight, how to study 14 hours in one day and much more.

At the moment you can get a free copy of

"33.5 Power Habits"!

Go and get it now!! At: ProjectSuperPerformance.com

Also! If you enjoyed this book check my other book named:

"Positive Thinking" Buy it by visiting

"www.amazon.com//dp/B014P7D654"

Or see the preview on next page first.

Preview from "*Positive Thinking*"

"I want to thank you and congratulate you for downloading the book, Positive Thinking.

This book contains proven steps and strategies on how to rid your life of all the negative thinking and destructive influences that do nothing but bring you down.

We all want to be happy in life, and as a general rule of thumb we do what we can to make our lives happy. We go to extremes to do things that will hopefully make us happy, whether it be buying things, going on exotic trips all over the world, dating, working, or whatever it may be, mankind is on a constant trek to gain happiness.

If you stop for a second and really give it some thought, you will see that I am right. Everything we do and say is for the hopeful end result that we will then be happy with our lives.

Maybe if we made more money we would be happy. Or maybe if we had more friends, maybe if you looked like that person or lost 5 pounds, then you would be happy.

I hate to be the one to say it, but ultimately those things have nothing to do with how happy you are. That is why you see people who are simply stunning to look at, have more money than they know what to do with, and all the comforts that you long for, yet they are still not happy.

What makes this seem even bleaker is the fact that there is no magic formula for happiness, you can't ever make the right number of anything to ensure you will be happy tomorrow. The newness wears off of any new relationship, things get old and break.

Even after a long vacation you have to deal with the stress of going back to work, figure out what you missed, what you need to do now, and how you are going to pay for everything you did when you were out and about in the world. And after all of this dies down, you start to feel overwhelmed about your life once again, then it isn't long before you are hoping to go on another vacation.

But this can't be it. There are a lot of happy people out there. Chances are, you know a few of them. They are those people that just go about life, and no matter what their situation is, they seem to be happy.

There doesn't seem to be a thing on this planet that is able to shake them. They are clearly the 'glass is always half-full' types, and it doesn't seem to matter if it is hot, cold, windy, rainy, sunny, or anything.

In fact, they may be dressed well, dressed poorly, rich, poor, struggling… who knows? Yet they always seem to be happy. It is almost as if you can't bring them down even if you tried.

Of course there are the other people in the world, too. Those that have everything handed to them, and have the most cushioned life that someone could ask for, yet nothing is ever good enough. They manage to find fault in everything, even if it is something they thought they wanted.

These people are everywhere, but they don't seem to have the same power as the positive thinkers. Those that are positive just seem to rise above the crowd and do their own thing, and not let themselves be bothered by what is going on with the rest of the world.

So what is their secret? How did they manage to reach this level of happiness, and is there a way you can get it for yourself? Do you have to be some sort of superhero to feel happy that often, or is there really something simple that you can learn to do that will help you to also be that happy?

Don't worry, these people are not superheroes, they have just figured out what it means to think positively. Positive thinking is powerful, and it changes how you view every aspect of your life.

No matter what you may be going through, there is always a reason to be happy, and thinking positively will help you achieve that.

By the time you reach the end of this book, you will be able to:

- *Think positively no matter what your situation is*
- *Find the good in everything*
- *Look up, and not down, when bad things happen*
- *And learn to apply this thinking to every aspect of your life*

No matter who you are or what you have been through, you will be able to also learn the art of positive thinking, and in no time at all you will notice a drastic... and positive... difference start to take root in your own life.

So what are you waiting for? There is a life of positive out there, just waiting for you to join in.

Thanks again for downloading this book, I hope you enjoy it!"

If you want to read more visit: www.amazon.com//dp/B014P7D654!

"Positive Thinking" have at the moment positive 60 reviews and 4.8/5 in ratings! 94pages of pure value. Available on both kindle and in paperback.

Here is one of the reviews, this one from Rick D:

"My favorite book so far on positive thinking and optimism thus far. Most books on positive thinking and optimism are not realistic and sometimes harmful. For example, thinking that everyone is nice and won't take advantage of you is the quickest way to getting taken advantage of. Most true positive thinkers (or what I like to call; practical optimists) realize bad things happen to them and those events can happen in the future, but a lot

of people are incredibly seeped into negativity, that it is also harmful. The solution is NOT to do a 180 degree change from negative thinking into nothing but positive thinking because that can also be detrimental. You must take the more difficult path of understanding when to be positive and to be practically pessimistic. This book goes into further detail on this subject and again, most people need this book since most people think negatively too much, even when they should be thinking more positively in a situation; for example, when something 'bad' happens to them, they should take it in stride and learn from it, rather than dwelling on the negative. Remember Thomas Edison had over 1,000 fails before creating the first lightbulb, and he learned from each of his 'failings.'"

And again, thank you for reading "Learning" Please leave a review by visiting: www.amazon.com//dp/B0161L2WES !

Thank You!

Cover Created By:

FreePik.com